BLEND ACTIVE

Recipe Book

Naturally Delicious Blend & Go Personal Blender
Smoothies for Workouts, Weight Loss
and Good Health

D1493894

MIMI COLLINS

ISBN-13: 978-1515008996
ISBN-10: 1515008991

CONTENTS

DRINK SMOOTHIES—YOUR BODY WILL LOVE IT!

Hi, I'm Mimi! I am here to tell you that drinking healthy smoothies is one of the easiest ways to improve your health and lose weight. I've created this smoothie book for people like you who want to improve your health—the easiest possible way. At first, when I started to make smoothies I wasn't very confident and I didn't think that I would last past my first smoothie. But like you, my motivation came from the fact that I wanted to find an easy way to improve my health, and so, I decided to stick with it. Before I started my daily smoothie regime, I ate every food on the planet. Furthermore, I weighed in at a whopping 15 stones (210 pounds). Even more, my cholesterol and my blood pressure was sky high.

Within my first three weeks of drinking just one smoothie as a meal replacement I had dropped 1 stone and lost about 3 inches. I also noticed that I had a tremendous increase in my energy level. By my eight week of smoothies, I felt like I could run a marathon. It was the best I'd felt in years, but the best was yet to come. Later, I got off my meds and I also lost another 37 pounds. Gradually, my habit of drinking daily smoothies had transformed my life and I was able to resolve much of my serious health issues. Then, one thing led to another. Eventually, I naturally became passionate about drinking smoothies and decided to share my passion with others. I wanted to help others experience restored health, vitality and weight loss—just like me.

Interestingly, these smoothies can work quickly! They are an amazingly helpful and fast way to improve your health. Very often, people can begin to see results within just a few days of starting a daily smoothie regime. Drinking balanced fruit and vegetable smoothies is one of the most soothing and effective ways to get lots of nutrients absorbed into your body in a short time. Consequently, these plant-based smoothies have been found to have consistently helped a lot of people to improve their health.

Everyone can enjoy these smoothies. I have compiled my most delicious and healthy recipes in this one complete book. My smoothies are tasty, easy-to-make, and loaded with vital nutrients. Now, everyone can enjoy the convenience and superb health benefits of these personal blender smoothies. Each new day presents an opportunity for you to transform your life—one smoothie at a time. Just choose a recipe, get the ingredients and have fun! Before you know it, you too will see and feel the difference.

MORNING SMOOTHIES

RASPBERRY BANANA PEAK

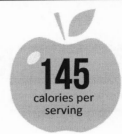

145 calories per serving

Ingredients

- ¼ cup (60ml) unsweetened Acai Berry Juice
- 1 Banana, peeled and sliced
- ½ cup (73g) fresh Raspberries
- 1 cup (67g) fresh Kale, trimmed and chopped
- 1 tablespoon Ground Flaxseeds
- ½-inch (1cm) Ginger Root, thinly sliced
- ½ cup (120ml) Purified Water

Directions

In a high speed blender or smoothie maker, add all of the ingredients.
Blend until smooth and enjoy.

NOTE

Adding more water will result in *thinner* smoothies while adding less water will result in *thicker* smoothies. You are encouraged to add water according to your personal preference for thicker or thinner smoothies.

ORANGE BERRY CREAM

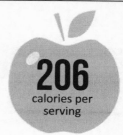

206 calories per serving

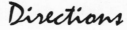

Ingredients

- ½ cup (120ml) fresh Orange Juice
- ½ cup (120ml) Nonfat Plain Greek Yogurt
- ½ cup (73g) fresh Mixed Berries
- 1 large fresh Plum, pitted and chopped
- ¼ teaspoon Ground Cinnamon
- 2 Ice Cubes

Directions

In a high speed blender or smoothie maker, add all of the ingredients.
Blend until smooth and enjoy.

CHERRY PLUM RIPPLE

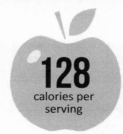

128
calories per
serving

Ingredients

- ½ cup (120ml) fresh/unsweetened Cherry Juice
- 1 large fresh Plum, pitted and chopped
- ½ cup fresh Cherries, pitted
- ½ inch (1cm) Ginger Root, thinly sliced
- 2 Ice Cubes
- ½ cup (120ml) Purified Water

Directions

In a high speed blender or smoothie maker, add all of the ingredients.
Blend until smooth and enjoy.

NOTE

Adding more water will result in *thinner* smoothies while adding less water will result in *thicker* smoothies. You are encouraged to add water according to your personal preference for thicker or thinner smoothies.

BANANA LIME PIE

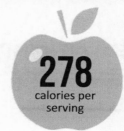

278
calories per
serving

Ingredients

- ½ cup (120ml) unsweetened Almond Milk
- ½ cup (120ml) Key Lime Greek Yogurt
- 1 Banana, peeled, sliced and frozen

- 3 large fresh Strawberries, hulled
- 1 tablespoon Ground Flaxseeds
- ½ scoop unsweetened Protein Powder
- 2 Ice Cubes

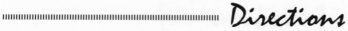

Directions

In a high speed blender or smoothie maker, add all of the ingredients.
Blend until smooth and enjoy.

SLIMMING STRAWBERRY PARADE

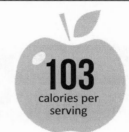

103 calories per serving

Ingredients

- ½ cup (120ml) unsweetened Almond Milk
- ½ cup (72g) fresh Strawberries, hulled and sliced
- ½ cup (70g) fresh Blueberries
- ½ cup (76g) fresh Watermelon, seeded and chopped
- ½ teaspoon Ground Cinnamon
- 2 Ice Cubes
- ½ cup (120ml) Purified Water

Directions

In a high speed blender or smoothie maker, add all of the ingredients. Blend until smooth and enjoy.

NOTE

Adding more water will result in *thinner* smoothies while adding less water will result in *thicker* smoothies. You are encouraged to add water according to your personal preference for thicker or thinner smoothies.

STRAWBERRY AVOCADO SPLIT

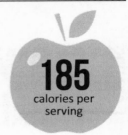

185
calories per serving

Ingredients

- ½ cup (120ml) unsweetened Almond Milk
- ¼ cup (60ml) Nonfat Plain Greek Yogurt
- ½ cups (72g) Strawberries, frozen

- 1 Medjool Date, pitted
- 1 slice (10g) Avocado, peeled and chopped
- 1 tablespoon Chia Seeds
- 2 Ice Cubes (optional)

Directions

In a high speed blender or smoothie maker, add all of the ingredients.
Blend until smooth and enjoy.

BLUEBERRY APPLE GLAZE

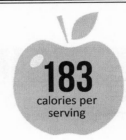

183 calories per serving

Ingredients

- ½ cup (120ml) unsweetened Organic Coconut Milk
- ½ cup (70g) fresh Blueberries
- ½ Banana, peeled and sliced
- 1 Gala Apple, peeled, cored and chopped

- 1 tablespoon Ground Flaxseeds
- 2 Ice Cubes (optional)
- ½ cup (120ml) Purified Water

Directions

In a high speed blender or smoothie maker, add all of the ingredients. Blend until smooth and enjoy.

NOTE

Adding more water will result in *thinner* smoothies while adding less water will result in *thicker* smoothies. You are encouraged to add water according to your personal preference for thicker or thinner smoothies.

BANANA BERRY PUDDING

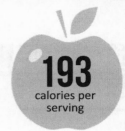

193
calories per serving

Ingredients

- ¼ cup (60ml) fresh Orange Juice
- ½ cup (120ml) Strawberry Greek Yogurt
- ½ cup (72g) Strawberries, hulled, sliced and frozen
- ¼ cup (37g) Blueberries, frozen
- ½ Banana, peeled and sliced
- ½ cup (120ml) Purified Water

Directions

In a high speed blender or smoothie maker, add all of the ingredients. Blend until smooth and enjoy.

NOTE

Adding more water will result in *thinner* smoothies while adding less water will result in *thicker* smoothies. You are encouraged to add water according to your personal preference for thicker or thinner smoothies.

ALMOND TROPICANA SWIZZLE

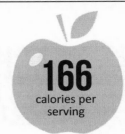

166 calories per serving

Ingredients

- ½ cup (120ml) unsweetened Almond Milk
- ½ tablespoon organic Almond Butter
- ¼ cup (47g) Mango Chunks, frozen

- ½ cup (83g) Pineapple Chunks, frozen
- 1 tablespoon Ground Flaxseeds
- ½ cup (120ml) Purified Water

Directions

In a high speed blender or smoothie maker, add all of the ingredients. Blend until smooth and enjoy.

NOTE

Adding more water will result in *thinner* smoothies while adding less water will result in *thicker* smoothies. You are encouraged to add water according to your personal preference for thicker or thinner smoothies.

PEACHY GRAPEFRUIT BLIZZARD

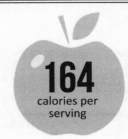

164 calories per serving

Ingredients

- ½ cup (120ml) fat-free plain Greek Yogurt
- ½ Grapefruit, peeled, seeded and sectioned
- ½ Banana, peeled and sliced
- 1 Peach, pitted and chopped
- 2 Ice Cubes
- ½ cup (120ml) Purified Water

Directions

In a high speed blender or smoothie maker, add all of the ingredients. Blend until smooth and enjoy.

NOTE

Adding more water will result in *thinner* smoothies while adding less water will result in *thicker* smoothies. You are encouraged to add water according to your personal preference for thicker or thinner smoothies.

3

GREEN CLEANSING SMOOTHIES

PEAR BRICKLE

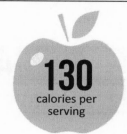

130
calories per
serving

Ingredients

- 1 Pear, peeled, cored and sliced
- ½ Banana, peeled and sliced
- ½ cup (30g) fresh Spinach

- ½-inch (1cm) Ginger Root, thinly sliced
- 1 cup (240ml) Purified Water

Directions

In a high speed blender or smoothie maker, add all of the ingredients.
Blend until smooth and enjoy.

NOTE

Adding more water will result in *thinner* smoothies while adding less water will result in *thicker* smoothies. You are encouraged to add water according to your personal preference for thicker or thinner smoothies.

AVOCADO KALE SWIRL

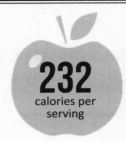

232 calories per serving

Ingredients

- 1 large Green Apple, peeled, cored and sliced
- 1 slice (10g) Avocado, peeled and chopped

- 1 Medjool Date, pitted
- 1 tablespoon Ground Flaxseeds
- ½ cup (34g) fresh Baby Kale
- 1 cup (240ml) Purified Water

Directions

In a high speed blender or smoothie maker, add all of the ingredients. Blend until smooth and enjoy.

NOTE

Adding more water will result in *thinner* smoothies while adding less water will result in *thicker* smoothies. You are encouraged to add water according to your personal preference for thicker or thinner smoothies.

MANGO KIWI PUNCH

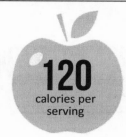

120 calories per serving

Ingredients

- 1 Kiwi, peeled and chopped
- ½ cup (14g) Romaine Lettuce, torn
- ½ cup (94g) Mango Chunks, frozen
- ½ tablespoon fresh Parsley Leaves
- ½-inch (1cm) Ginger Root, thinly sliced
- 1 cup (240ml) Purified Water

Directions

In a high speed blender or smoothie maker, add all of the ingredients. Blend until smooth and enjoy.

NOTE

Adding more water will result in *thinner* smoothies while adding less water will result in *thicker* smoothies. You are encouraged to add water according to your personal preference for thicker or thinner smoothies.

GREEN BERRY MELLO

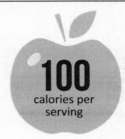

100
calories per
serving

Ingredients

- ½ cup (72g) Strawberries, hulled, sliced and frozen
- ¼ cup (23g) seedless Grapes
- ½ cup (34g) fresh Kale, trimmed and chopped
- 1 tablespoon Ground Flaxseeds
- 1 cup (240ml) Purified Water

Directions

In a high speed blender or smoothie maker, add all of the ingredients.
Blend until smooth and enjoy.

NOTE

Adding more water will result in *thinner* smoothies while adding less water will result in *thicker* smoothies. You are encouraged to add water according to your personal preference for thicker or thinner smoothies.

PEACH SPRING MINT

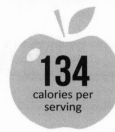

134 calories per serving

Ingredients

- 1 Peach, pitted and chopped
- 1 Medjool Date, pitted
- ½ small Cucumber, peeled and chopped
- ½ cup (28g) fresh Spring Greens, chopped
- ½ tablespoon fresh Mint Leaves
- 1 cup (240ml) Purified Water

Directions

In a high speed blender or smoothie maker, add all of the ingredients. Blend until smooth and enjoy.

NOTE

Adding more water will result in *thinner* smoothies while adding less water will result in *thicker* smoothies. You are encouraged to add water according to your personal preference for thicker or thinner smoothies.

RASPY DANDY FUDGE

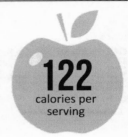

122 calories per serving

Ingredients

- ½ cup (73g) fresh Raspberries
- 1 slice (10g) Avocado, peeled and chopped
- 1 cup (27g) Romaine Lettuce, torn
- 1 Medjool Date, pitted
- 2 Ice Cubes
- 1 cup (240ml) Purified Water

Directions

In a high speed blender or smoothie maker, add all of the ingredients. Blend until smooth and enjoy.

NOTE

Adding more water will result in *thinner* smoothies while adding less water will result in *thicker* smoothies. You are encouraged to add water according to your personal preference for thicker or thinner smoothies.

BLUEBERRY GREEN COBBLER

173 calories per serving

Ingredients

- ½ cup (36g) Green Cabbage, chopped
- ½ small Green Bell Pepper, seeded and chopped
- ½ cup (94g) Mango Chunks, frozen
- ½ cup (70g) fresh Blueberries
- 1 Medjool Date, pitted
- 1 cup (240ml) Purified Water

Directions

In a high speed blender or smoothie maker, add all of the ingredients. Blend until smooth and enjoy.

NOTE

Adding more water will result in *thinner* smoothies while adding less water will result in *thicker* smoothies. You are encouraged to add water according to your personal preference for thicker or thinner smoothies.

MIXED GREEN APPLE

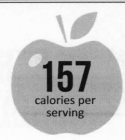

157
calories per
serving

Ingredients

- 1 Green Apple, peeled, cored and sliced
- ½ cup (72g) fresh Blackberries
- ½ cup (34g) fresh Baby Kale
- ½ cup (27g) Romaine Lettuce, chopped

- ½-inch (1cm) Ginger Root, thinly sliced
- ½ cup (120ml) Organic Coconut Water
- ½ cup (120ml) Purified Water

Directions

In a high speed blender or smoothie maker, add all of the ingredients. Blend until smooth and enjoy.

NOTE

Adding more water will result in *thinner* smoothies while adding less water will result in *thicker* smoothies. You are encouraged to add water according to your personal preference for thicker or thinner smoothies.

CREAMY STRAWBERRY CHASER

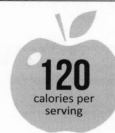

120 calories per serving

Ingredients

- 1 large fresh Plum, pitted and chopped
- ½ cups (72g) Strawberries, hulled and sliced
- 1 slice (10g) Avocado, peeled and chopped
- ½ cup (15g) fresh Spinach
- 1 tablespoon Ground Flaxseeds
- ½ cup (120ml) organic Coconut Water
- ½ cup (120ml) Purified Water

Directions

In a high speed blender or smoothie maker, add all of the ingredients. Blend until smooth and enjoy.

NOTE

Adding more water will result in *thinner* smoothies while adding less water will result in *thicker* smoothies. You are encouraged to add water according to your personal preference for thicker or thinner smoothies.

DELUXE CARROT MEDLEY

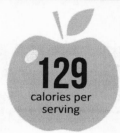

129
calories per
serving

Ingredients

- 1 medium Orange, peeled, seeded and chopped
- ½ cup (113g) fresh Cherries, pitted
- ½ cup (34g) fresh Baby Kale
- ¼ cup (28g) Carrots, peeled and chopped
- 2 Ice Cubes
- ¾ cup (180m) Purified Water

Directions

In a high speed blender or smoothie maker, add all of the ingredients.
Blend until smooth and enjoy.

NOTE

Adding more water will result in *thinner* smoothies while adding less water will result in *thicker* smoothies. You are encouraged to add water according to your personal preference for thicker or thinner smoothies.

4

ANTI-AGING SMOOTHIES

YOUTH CODE BOOGIE

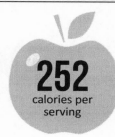

252 calories per serving

Ingredients

- ½ cup (15g) fresh Spinach
- 1 Banana, peeled and sliced
- 1 slice (10g) Avocado, peeled and chopped
- ½ cup (73g) Blueberries, frozen
- ½ tablespoon extra-virgin Organic Coconut Oil

- ½ cup (120ml) unsweetened Almond Milk
- 1 tablespoon Ground Flaxseeds
- ½ cup (120ml) Purified Water

Directions

In a high speed blender or smoothie maker, add all of the ingredients. Blend until smooth and enjoy.

NOTE

Adding more water will result in *thinner* smoothies while adding less water will result in *thicker* smoothies. You are encouraged to add water according to your personal preference for thicker or thinner smoothies.

VITAMIN C ELIXIR

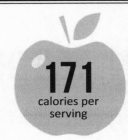

171
calories per
serving

Ingredients

- ½ cup (72g) fresh Strawberries, hulled and sliced
- ½ cup (70g) fresh Blueberries
- ½ cup (120ml) Nonfat Plain Greek Yogurt

- 1 tablespoon Chia Seeds
- ½ tablespoon fresh Mint Leaves
- ¼ cup (60ml) unsweetened Cherry Juice
- ½ cup (120ml) Purified Water

Directions

In a high speed blender or smoothie maker, add all of the ingredients.
Blend until smooth and enjoy.

NOTE

Adding more water will result in *thinner* smoothies while adding less water will result in *thicker* smoothies. You are encouraged to add water according to your personal preference for thicker or thinner smoothies.

BETA SKIN SERUM

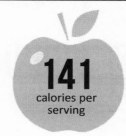

141
calories per
serving

Ingredients

- ½ cup (34g) fresh Baby Kale
- ¼ cup (28g) Carrots, peeled and chopped
- ½ cup (94g) Mango Chunks, frozen
- 1 tablespoon Chia Seeds
- ¼ cup (600ml) unsweetened Organic Apple Juice
- ½ cup (120ml) Purified Water

Directions

In a high speed blender or smoothie maker, add all of the ingredients. Blend until smooth and enjoy.

NOTE

Adding more water will result in *thinner* smoothies while adding less water will result in *thicker* smoothies. You are encouraged to add water according to your personal preference for thicker or thinner smoothies.

WRINKLE AWAY BLISS

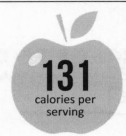

131 calories per serving

Ingredients

- ½ cup (94g) Mango Chunks, frozen
- ¼ cup (42g) Pineapple Chunks, frozen
- ½ small Cucumber, peeled and chopped
- ½ cup (28g) fresh Spring Greens, chopped
- ½ inch (1cm) Ginger Root, thinly sliced
- 1 tablespoon Ground Flaxseeds
- 1 cup (240ml) Purified Water

Directions

In a high speed blender or smoothie maker, add all of the ingredients. Blend until smooth and enjoy.

NOTE

Adding more water will result in *thinner* smoothies while adding less water will result in *thicker* smoothies. You are encouraged to add water according to your personal preference for thicker or thinner smoothies.

ANTIOXIDANT STRAWBERRY THRILL

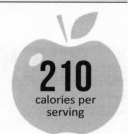

210 calories per serving

Ingredients

- 1 Banana, peeled and sliced
- ½ cup (72g) fresh Strawberries, hulled and sliced
- 1 slice (10g) Avocado, peeled and chopped

- 1 tablespoon Organic Cocoa Powder
- 1 tablespoon Chia Seeds
- 1 teaspoon Vanilla Extract
- 1 cup (240ml) Purified Water

Directions

In a high speed blender or smoothie maker, add all of the ingredients. Blend until smooth and enjoy.

NOTE

Adding more water will result in *thinner* smoothies while adding less water will result in *thicker* smoothies. You are encouraged to add water according to your personal preference for thicker or thinner smoothies.

ORANGE BERRY REFRESHER

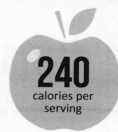

240 calories per serving

Ingredients

- ½ cup (73g) fresh Raspberries
- ½ cup (73g) Blueberries, frozen
- ½ medium Orange, peeled, seeded and chopped
- 1 Banana, peeled and sliced

- 1 tablespoon Ground Flaxseeds
- ¼ cup (60ml) Nonfat Plain Greek Yogurt
- 2 Ice cubes
- ½ cup (120ml) Purified Water

Directions

In a high speed blender or smoothie maker, add all of the ingredients. Blend until smooth and enjoy.

NOTE

Adding more water will result in *thinner* smoothies while adding less water will result in *thicker* smoothies. You are encouraged to add water according to your personal preference for thicker or thinner smoothies.

STRESS BUSTER BLAST

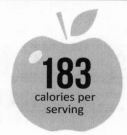

183 calories per serving

Ingredients

- ½ cup (15g) fresh Spinach
- ½ cup (34g) fresh Baby Kale
- 1 Pear, peeled, cored and sliced
- ½ cup (83g) Pineapple Chunks, frozen
- 1 teaspoon Organic Sunflower Oil
- 1 cup (240ml) Purified Water

Directions

In a high speed blender or smoothie maker, add all of the ingredients.
Blend until smooth and enjoy.

NOTE

Adding more water will result in *thinner* smoothies while adding less water will result in *thicker* smoothies. You are encouraged to add water according to your personal preference for thicker or thinner smoothies.

SKIN NOURISHING CRUMBLE

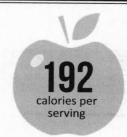

192 calories per serving

Ingredients

- ¼ cup (60ml) unsweetened Organic Coconut Milk
- ½ cup (113g) fresh Cherries, pitted
- ½ Banana, peeled and sliced
- 1 Gala Apple, peeled, cored and chopped

- 1 tablespoon Chia Seeds
- 1 teaspoon Vanilla Extract
- ½ teaspoon Ground Cinnamon
- 2 Ice Cubes
- ¾ cup (180ml) Purified Water

Directions

In a high speed blender or smoothie maker, add all of the ingredients.
Blend until smooth and enjoy.

NOTE

Adding more water will result in *thinner* smoothies while adding less water will result in *thicker* smoothies. You are encouraged to add water according to your personal preference for thicker or thinner smoothies.

ANTI-INFLAMMATORY CREAM BERRY

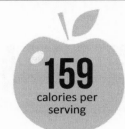

159 calories per serving

Ingredients

- 1 Peach, pitted and chopped
- 1 slice (10g) Avocado, peeled and chopped
- 1 cup (140g) fresh Blueberries
- ½ cup (120ml) Organic Pomegranate Juice

- 1 tablespoon Ground Flaxseeds =
- 2 Ice Cubes
- ½ cup (120ml) Purified Water

Directions

In a high speed blender or smoothie maker, add all of the ingredients. Blend until smooth and enjoy.

NOTE

Adding more water will result in *thinner* smoothies while adding less water will result in *thicker* smoothies. You are encouraged to add water according to your personal preference for thicker or thinner smoothies.

COLLAGEN BERRY FIX

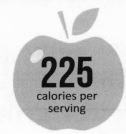

225 calories per serving

Ingredients

- ½ cup (72g) fresh Strawberries, hulled and sliced 38
- ½ cup (73g) fresh Raspberries 32
- ½ cup (94g) Mango Chunks, frozen 67
- ½ cup (33g) fresh Baby Kale – 17

- ½ cup (120ml) unsweetened Almond Milk 20
- ½ tablespoon organic Almond Butter 51
- ½ cup (120ml) Purified Water

Directions

In a high speed blender or smoothie maker, add all of the ingredients.
Blend until smooth and enjoy.

NOTE

Adding more water will result in *thinner* smoothies while adding less water will result in *thicker* smoothies. You are encouraged to add water according to your personal preference for thicker or thinner smoothies.

5

HEART HEALTHY SMOOTHIES

ARTERIES BERRY CLEANSER

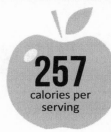

257
calories per
serving

Ingredients

- ½ cup (72g) fresh Strawberries, hulled and sliced
- 1 Banana, peeled and sliced
- ¼ cup (42g) Pineapple Chunks, frozen
- ½ cup (120ml) Nonfat Plain Greek Yogurt

- 1 tablespoon Chia Seeds
- ¼ cup (60ml) Organic Pomegranate Juice
- ½ cup (120ml) Purified Water

Directions

In a high speed blender or smoothie maker, add all of the ingredients.
Blend until smooth and enjoy.

NOTE

Adding more water will result in *thinner* smoothies while adding less water will result in *thicker* smoothies. You are encouraged to add water according to your personal preference for thicker or thinner smoothies.

THE HEART'S FRIEND

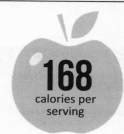

168 calories per serving

Ingredients

- ½ cup (34g) fresh Baby Kale
- ½ Banana, peeled and sliced
- ½ cup (94g) Mango Chunks, frozen
- 2 tablespoon Ground Flaxseeds

- ½ cup (120ml) Organic Coconut Water
- ½ cup (120ml) Purified Water

Directions

In a high speed blender or smoothie maker, add all of the ingredients.
Blend until smooth and enjoy.

NOTE

Adding more water will result in *thinner* smoothies while adding less water will result in *thicker* smoothies. You are encouraged to add water according to your personal preference for thicker or thinner smoothies.

STRESS BUSTER COCKTAIL

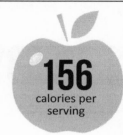

156 calories per serving

Ingredients

- ½ cup (14g) Romaine Lettuce, torn
- ½ cup (84g) Pineapple Chunks, frozen
- ½ cup (72g) fresh Blackberries
- ¼ cup (60ml) Reduced-fat Cottage Cheese
- 1 tablespoon Ground Flaxseeds
- ¼ cup (60ml) unsweetened Organic Apple Juice
- ¾ cup (180ml) Purified Water

Directions

In a high speed blender or smoothie maker, add all of the ingredients.
Blend until smooth and enjoy.

NOTE

Adding more water will result in *thinner* smoothies while adding less water will result in *thicker* smoothies. You are encouraged to add water according to your personal preference for thicker or thinner smoothies.

MERRY AVOCADO TONER

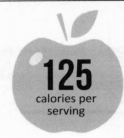

125
calories per serving

Ingredients

- ½ cup (120ml) unsweetened Almond Milk
- ½ cup (34g) fresh Baby Kale
- 1 slice (10g) Avocado, peeled and chopped

- ½ cup (46g) seedless Grapes
- 1 tablespoon Ground Flaxseeds
- ½ cup (120ml) Purified Water

Directions

In a high speed blender or smoothie maker, add all of the ingredients. Blend until smooth and enjoy.

NOTE

Adding more water will result in *thinner* smoothies while adding less water will result in *thicker* smoothies. You are encouraged to add water according to your personal preference for thicker or thinner smoothies.

HEARTY FRUIT PLEASER

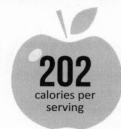

202 calories per serving

Ingredients

- ¼ cup (23g) seedless Grapes
- 1 Gala Apple, peeled, cored and chopped
- ½ cup (70g) fresh Blueberries
- ½ cup (72g) fresh Strawberries, hulled and sliced
- ¼ cup (60ml) fresh/unsweetened Cherry Juice
- 2 Ice Cubes
- ½ cup (120ml) Purified Water

Directions

In a high speed blender or smoothie maker, add all of the ingredients. Blend until smooth and enjoy.

NOTE

Adding more water will result in *thinner* smoothies while adding less water will result in *thicker* smoothies. You are encouraged to add water according to your personal preference for thicker or thinner smoothies.

ROMAINE BLUEBERRY BEAT

175 calories per serving

Ingredients

- ½ cup (14g) Romaine Lettuce, torn
- ½ cup (70g) fresh Blueberries
- 1 Banana, peeled and sliced
- ½ cup (120ml) Nonfat Blueberry Greek Yogurt
- 2 Ice Cubes
- ½ cup (120ml) Purified Water

Directions

In a high speed blender or smoothie maker, add all of the ingredients.
Blend until smooth and enjoy.

NOTE

Adding more water will result in *thinner* smoothies while adding less water will result in *thicker* smoothies. You are encouraged to add water according to your personal preference for thicker or thinner smoothies.

COMFORTING OAT SIZZLE

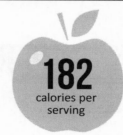

182 calories per serving

Ingredients

- ¼ cup (20g) Rolled Oats
- ½ Banana, peeled and sliced
- ½ cup (70g) fresh Blueberries
- ¾ cup (180ml) unsweetened Almond Milk
- ½ tablespoon Ground Flaxseeds
- 1 teaspoon Vanilla Extract
- ½ teaspoon Ground Cinnamon
- 2 Ice Cubes

Directions

In a high speed blender or smoothie maker, add all of the ingredients.
Blend until smooth and enjoy.

SUPERFOOD ACAI TONIC

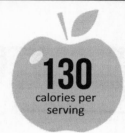

130
calories per serving

Ingredients

- 2 tablespoons organic Acai Berry Juice
- ½ cup (72g) fresh Raspberries
- ½ cup (94g) Mango Chunks, frozen

- 1 tablespoon Chia Seeds
- 2 Ice Cubes
- ¾ cup (180ml) Purified Water

Directions

In a high speed blender or smoothie maker, add all of the ingredients.
Blend until smooth and enjoy.

NOTE

Adding more water will result in *thinner* smoothies while adding less water will result in *thicker* smoothies. You are encouraged to add water according to your personal preference for thicker or thinner smoothies.

BEET REBOUND JUICE

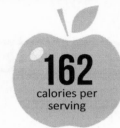

162
calories per
serving

Ingredients

- 1 small Beet, trimmed, peeled and chopped
- ¼ cup (28g) Carrots, peeled and chopped
- ½ cup (94g) Mango Chunks, frozen
- ¾ cup (180ml) unsweetened Almond Milk
- 1 tablespoon Ground Flaxseeds
- 1 teaspoon Vanilla Extract
- 2 Ice Cubes

Directions

In a high speed blender or smoothie maker, add all of the ingredients.
Blend until smooth and enjoy.

REFRESHING APPLE FRENZY

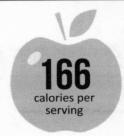

166 calories per serving

Ingredients

- 1 large Green Apple, peeled, cored and sliced
- 1 cup (36g) Swiss Chard, trimmed and chopped
- ½ cup (83g) Pineapple Chunks, frozen
- ½ tablespoon Lemon Juice
- 2 Ice Cubes
- 1 cup (240ml) Purified Water

Directions

In a high speed blender or smoothie maker, add all of the ingredients. Blend until smooth and enjoy.

NOTE

Adding more water will result in *thinner* smoothies while adding less water will result in *thicker* smoothies. You are encouraged to add water according to your personal preference for thicker or thinner smoothies.

6

HIGH ENERGY SMOOTHIES

BLUEBERRY POWER-UP

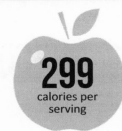

299
calories per
serving

Ingredients

- 1 Banana, peeled and sliced
- ½ cup (70g) fresh Blueberries
- 1 cup (67g) fresh Baby Kale
- ½ tablespoon organic Almond Butter

- ¼ cup (20g) Rolled Oats
- ¼ cup (60ml) unsweetened Organic Apple Juice
- ¾ cup (180ml) Purified Water

Directions

In a high speed blender or smoothie maker, add all of the ingredients.
Blend until smooth and enjoy.

NOTE

Adding more water will result in *thinner* smoothies while adding less water will result in *thicker* smoothies. You are encouraged to add water according to your personal preference for thicker or thinner smoothies.

MIXED ENERGY SWIRL

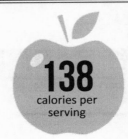

138
calories per
serving

Ingredients

- ½ cup (83g) Pineapple Chunks, frozen
- ½ cup (76g) fresh Watermelon, seeded and chopped
- ½ cup (70g) fresh Blueberries
- ½ cup (15g) fresh Spinach
- 1 tablespoon Ground Flaxseeds
- ¾ cup (180ml) Organic Coconut Water

Directions

In a high speed blender or smoothie maker, add all of the ingredients. Blend until smooth and enjoy.

KIWI GREEN GIANT

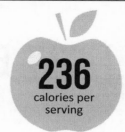

236
calories per
serving

Ingredients

- 1 Banana, peeled and sliced
- 1 Kiwi, peeled and chopped
- ½ cup (94g) Mango Chunks, frozen
- ½ cup (14g) Romaine Lettuce, torn
- ¾ cup (180ml) unsweetened Almond Milk
- 2 Ice Cubes

Directions

In a high speed blender or smoothie maker, add all of the ingredients.
Blend until smooth and enjoy.

CHIA BANANA GOODNESS

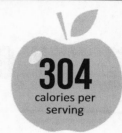

304 calories per serving

Ingredients

- 1 Banana, peeled and sliced
- 1 Pear, peeled, cored and sliced
- ¼ cup (23g) seedless Grapes
- ½ cup (15g) fresh Spinach
- 1 tablespoon Chia Seeds

- ½ tablespoon Organic Cocoa Powder
- ½ cup (120ml) Nonfat Greek Yogurt (use your favorite flavor)
- ¾ cup (180ml) Purified Water

Directions

In a high speed blender or smoothie maker, add all of the ingredients.
Blend until smooth and enjoy.

NOTE

Adding more water will result in *thinner* smoothies while adding less water will result in *thicker* smoothies. You are encouraged to add water according to your personal preference for thicker or thinner smoothies.

CHERRY GALA FIESTA

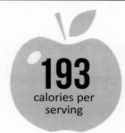

193 calories per serving

Ingredients

- ½ cup (70g) fresh Blueberries
- 1 Gala Apple, peeled, cored and chopped
- 1 cup (67g) fresh Baby Kale
- ¼ cup (60ml) fresh/unsweetened Cherry Juice
- ¼ cup (60ml) unsweetened Almond Milk
- 1 tablespoon Ground Flaxseeds
- 2 Ice Cubes

Directions

In a high speed blender or smoothie maker, add all of the ingredients.
Blend until smooth and enjoy.

PEACHY ORANGE MIST

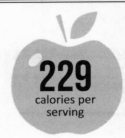

229 calories per serving

Ingredients

- 1 medium Peach, pitted and chopped
- 1 small Banana, peeled and sliced
- ¼ cup (60ml) Nonfat Plain Greek Yogurt
- 1 tablespoon Ground Flaxseeds
- ½ cup (120ml) fresh Orange Juice
- 2 Ice Cubes

Directions

In a high speed blender or smoothie maker, add all of the ingredients. Blend until smooth and enjoy.

JAZZY HONEYDEW MELON

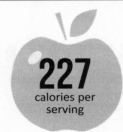

227 calories per serving

Ingredients

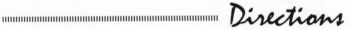

- 1 Kiwi, peeled and chopped
- 1 cup (152g) Honeydew Melon, peeled and chopped
- ½-inch (1cm) Ginger Root, thinly sliced

- ¾ cup (180ml) unsweetened Organic Apple Juice
- 1 tablespoon Ground Flaxseeds
- 2 Ice Cubes

Directions

In a high speed blender or smoothie maker, add all of the ingredients.
Blend until smooth and enjoy.

PINEAPPLE BRICKLE

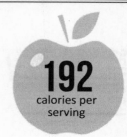

192
calories per
serving

Ingredients

- ½ cup (83g) Pineapple Chunks, frozen
- 1 Banana, peeled and sliced
- ½ cup (72g) fresh Blackberries
- 1 tablespoon Chia Seeds
- ¾ cup (180ml) Almond Milk
- 2 Ice Cubes

Directions

In a high speed blender or smoothie maker, add all of the ingredients.
Blend until smooth and enjoy.

STRAWBERRY JIGGLES

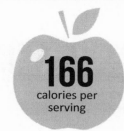

166
calories per serving

Ingredients

- ¼ cup (60ml) Organic Pomegranate Juice
- ½ cup (72g) fresh Strawberries, hulled and sliced
- ½ Banana, peeled and sliced
- ½ cup (28g) fresh Spring Greens, chopped
- 1 tablespoon Ground Flaxseeds
- ¼ cup (60ml) Nonfat Plain Greek Yogurt
- 2 Ice Cubes
- ½ cup (120ml) Purified Water

Directions

In a high speed blender or smoothie maker, add all of the ingredients. Blend until smooth and enjoy.

NOTE

Adding more water will result in *thinner* smoothies while adding less water will result in *thicker* smoothies. You are encouraged to add water according to your personal preference for thicker or thinner smoothies.

BLAZING MANGO BERRY

115 calories per serving

Ingredients

- ¼ cup (60ml) unsweetened Organic Coconut Milk
- ½ cup (94g) Mango Chunks, frozen
- ½ cup (73g) fresh Mixed Berries (use your favorites)

- ½ cup (15g) fresh Spinach
- ¾ cup (180ml) Purified Water

Directions

In a high speed blender or smoothie maker, add all of the ingredients. Blend until smooth and enjoy.

NOTE

Adding more water will result in *thinner* smoothies while adding less water will result in *thicker* smoothies. You are encouraged to add water according to your personal preference for thicker or thinner smoothies.

EVERYDAY SMOOTHIES

BANANA BERRY VELVET

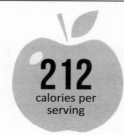

212
calories per
serving

Ingredients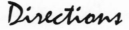

- ½ cup (120ml) Almond Milk, unsweetened
- 1 medium Banana, frozen
- ½ cup (73g) fresh Raspberries
- ½ tablespoon Almond Butter
- ½ tablespoon Protein Powder, unsweetened
- ¼ teaspoon Vanilla Extract
- ¼ cup (60ml) Purified Water
- 2 Ice Cubes

Directions

In a high speed blender or smoothie maker, add all of the ingredients.
Blend until smooth and enjoy.

CHIA PINADA

125 calories per serving

Ingredients

- ¼ cup (60ml) unsweetened Almond Milk
- ¼ cup (60ml) unsweetened Organic Coconut Milk
- ½ cup (94g) Mango Chunks, frozen
- ¼ cup (42g) Pineapple Chunks, frozen
- 1 tablespoon Chia Seeds
- 2 Ice Cubes
- ½ cup (120ml) Purified Water

Directions

In a high speed blender or smoothie maker, add all of the ingredients.
Blend until smooth and enjoy.

NOTE

Adding more water will result in *thinner* smoothies while adding less water will result in *thicker* smoothies. You are encouraged to add water according to your personal preference for thicker or thinner smoothies.

MANGO GREEN MIX

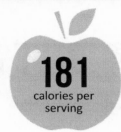

181 calories per serving

Ingredients

- ½ cup (120ml) unsweetened Almond Milk
- ½ cup (120ml) Nonfat Blueberry Greek Yogurt (or use your favorite flavor)
- ½ cup (94g) Mango, frozen, peeled, pitted and chopped
- 1 tablespoon Ground Flaxseeds
- ½ cup (15g) fresh Spinach
- ½ cup (34g) fresh Baby Kale
- 2 Ice Cubes

Directions

In a high speed blender or smoothie maker, add all of the ingredients. Blend until smooth and enjoy.

BLUE ALMOND BUNNY

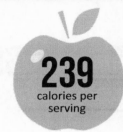

239
calories per
serving

Ingredients

- ½ cup (120ml) unsweetened Almond Milk
- 1 cup (140g) fresh Blueberries
- 1 Medjool Date, pitted
- ½ tablespoon Almond Butter

- ½ tablespoon Protein Powder, unsweetened
- 2 Ice Cubes
- ½ cup (120ml) Purified Water

Directions

In a high speed blender or smoothie maker, add all of the ingredients.
Blend until smooth and enjoy.

NOTE

Adding more water will result in *thinner* smoothies while adding less water will result in *thicker* smoothies. You are encouraged to add water according to your personal preference for thicker or thinner smoothies.

PEAR DELIGHT

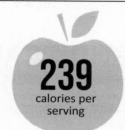

239
calories per
serving

Ingredients

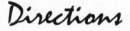

- ½ cup (120ml) unsweetened Almond Milk
- ¼ cup (60ml) plain Greek Yogurt, fat-free
- 1 Pear, peeled, cored and sliced
- 1 Medjool Date, pitted and chopped

- ½ tablespoon Organic Cocoa Powder
- 1 tablespoon Chia Seeds
- Pinch of Ground Cinnamon
- 2 Ice Cubes

Directions

In a high speed blender or smoothie maker, add all of the ingredients.
Blend until smooth and enjoy.

PINEAPPLE CHERRY CICLE

217 calories per serving

Ingredients

- ½ cup (120ml) unsweetened Almond Milk
- 1 slice (10g) Avocado, peeled and chopped
- ½ cup (83g) Pineapple Chunks, frozen
- 1 cup (225g) fresh Cherries, pitted
- 1 Medjool Date, pitted (optional)
- ½ cup (120ml) Purified Water

Directions

In a high speed blender or smoothie maker, add all of the ingredients. Blend until smooth and enjoy.

NOTE

Adding more water will result in *thinner* smoothies while adding less water will result in *thicker* smoothies. You are encouraged to add water according to your personal preference for thicker or thinner smoothies.

GINGER CARROT ENERGY

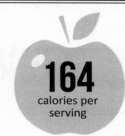

164 calories per serving

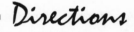

Ingredients

- ¾ cup (180ml) brewed and cooled Green Tea
- ½ cup (94g) Mango, frozen and chopped
- 1 Medjool Date, pitted
- ¼ cup (28g) Carrots, peeled and chopped

- ½-inch (1cm) Ginger Root, thinly sliced
- 1 tablespoon Chia Seeds
- 2 Ice Cubes

Directions

In a high speed blender or smoothie maker, add all of the ingredients. Blend until smooth and enjoy.

COOLING PEACH FIX

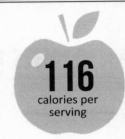

116
calories per
serving

Ingredients

- ½ cup (120ml) Organic Coconut Water
- 1 Peach, pitted and chopped
- ½ small Cucumber, peeled and chopped

- 1 tablespoon Ground Flaxseeds
- ½ tablespoon Nut Butter (use your favourite)
- 2 Ice Cubes
- ½ cup (120ml) Purified Water

Directions

In a high speed blender or smoothie maker, add all of the ingredients. Blend until smooth and enjoy.

NOTE

Adding more water will result in *thinner* smoothies while adding less water will result in *thicker* smoothies. You are encouraged to add water according to your personal preference for thicker or thinner smoothies.

STRAWBERRY CRAN CREEK

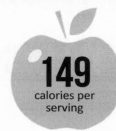

149
calories per serving

Ingredients

- ¼ cup (60ml) fresh Cranberry juice
- ½ cup (120ml) Nonfat Greek Yogurt (use your favorite flavor)
- ½ cup (72g) fresh Strawberries, hulled and sliced
- 1 cup (27g) Romaine Lettuce, torn
- 1 tablespoon Ground Flaxseeds
- 2 Ice Cubes
- ½ cup (120ml) Purified Water

Directions

In a high speed blender or smoothie maker, add all of the ingredients. Blend until smooth and enjoy.

NOTE

Adding more water will result in *thinner* smoothies while adding less water will result in *thicker* smoothies. You are encouraged to add water according to your personal preference for thicker or thinner smoothies.

APRICOT GREEN GLORY

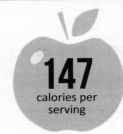

147
calories per
serving

Ingredients

- ½ cup (120ml) unsweetened Almond Milk
- 1 Gala Apple, peeled, cored and chopped
- ½ cup (76g) Apricots, pitted and chopped

- 1 cup (55g) fresh Spring Greens, chopped
- 2 Ice Cubes
- ½ cup (120ml) Purified Water

Directions

In a high speed blender or smoothie maker, add all of the ingredients.
Blend until smooth and enjoy.

NOTE

Adding more water will result in *thinner* smoothies while adding less water will result in *thicker* smoothies. You are encouraged to add water according to your personal preference for thicker or thinner smoothies.

DUNKIN KALE CREEK

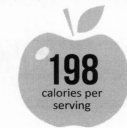

198
calories per
serving

Ingredients

- ½ tablespoon Lemon Juice
- 1 Green Apple, peeled, cored and sliced
- ½ Banana, peeled and sliced

- ¼ cup (47g) Mango Chunks, frozen
- ½ cup (33g) fresh Baby Kale
- 1 tablespoon Ground Flaxseeds
- 1 cup (240ml) Purified Water

Directions

In a high speed blender or smoothie maker, add all of the ingredients.
Blend until smooth and enjoy.

NOTE

Adding more water will result in *thinner* smoothies while adding less water will result in *thicker* smoothies. You are encouraged to add water according to your personal preference for thicker or thinner smoothies.

PUMPKIN PEAR PIXIE

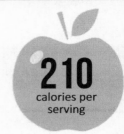

210 calories per serving

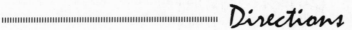

Ingredients

- ¾ cup (180ml) unsweetened Almond Milk
- ¼ cup (62g) homemade Pumpkin Puree
- 1 Medjool Date, pitted

- 1 Pear, peeled, cored and sliced
- 1 tablespoon Ground Flaxseeds
- ½ teaspoon Pumpkin Pie Spice
- ½ teaspoon Ground Cinnamon
- Pinch of Salt (optional)

Directions

In a high speed blender or smoothie maker, add all of the ingredients. Blend until smooth and enjoy.

GLOW AND SHOW

Unfortunately, most of us have been brain washed into thinking that to look great and feel great we have to break the bank. But that couldn't be further from the truth. Looking great and feeling great is quite an attainable goal and it doesn't have to be expensive.

My never-ending gratitude for discovering that I could change my life by drinking smoothies is indescribable. Each day I continue to improve and maintain good health and it keeps getting better and better. Best of all, making smoothies is easy. I don't have to count calories, I don't have to starve myself and I don't have to engage in a rigorous workout. I simply make and enjoy my smoothie. What I have done is to simply replace one of my main meals with a single serving of smoothie each day. That's all and I don't get overburdened by it.

It's indeed a pleasure to share my smoothies with you and countless others so that everyone can enjoy the results and freedom that comes with being healthy. Just make these smoothies a part of your daily diet and soon you'll experience exactly what it feels like to truly glow and show—being healthy from the inside out.

Thanks again for purchasing my smoothie recipe book. I'll be thrilled if you would let other readers know about your experience in consistently drinking smoothies.

Live Happy and Healthy,
Mimi Collins

Printed in Great Britain
by Amazon.co.uk, Ltd.,
Marston Gate.